SYNDROME X
AND
SX-FRACTION

A Breakthrough for the Deadly Quartet (Diabetes, Obesity, Hypertension and High Cholesterol) Which Affects More than 60 Million Americans

Mark Kaylor, Ph.D.
AND Ken Babal, C.N.

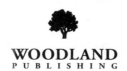

WOODLAND
PUBLISHING

For order information or other inquiries, please contact us:
Woodland Publishing
448 East 800 North
Orem, Utah
84097
Visit us at our web site: www.woodlandpublishing.com
or call us toll-free: (800) 777-2665

The information in this book is for educational purposes only and is not recommended as a means of diagnosing or treating an illness. All matters concerning physical and mental health should be supervised by a health practitioner knowledgeable in treating that particular condition. Neither the publisher nor the author directly or indirectly dispenses medical advice, nor do they prescribe any remedies or assume any responsibility for those who choose to treat themselves.

ISBN 1-58054-373-1
Printed in the United States of America

Contents

Contents

Syndrome X

1) WHAT IS IT?

It sounds like it could be the name of a science fiction movie, but Syndrome X is actually a term for a cluster of disease-causing conditions including high blood pressure, high triglycerides (blood fats), decreased high density lipoproteins (HDL, the "good cholesterol"), abdominal obesity and insulin resistance which tend to appear together. Some doctors make the diagnosis if a person has two or more of the symptoms. About one out of every four Americans, or more than 60 million people in this country, has some degree of Syndrome X, which sets the stage for type 2 diabetes, heart disease and other life-threatening diseases. Unfortunately, most of us are not aware of this *sweeping American epidemic*.

Syndrome X, also called as Metabolic Syndrome, Insulin Resistance Syndrome or the Deadly Quartet, develops over the years as the result of consuming far too many refined sugars and carbohydrates combined with a sedentary lifestyle of little or no exercise. The result is that we have constantly elevated levels of blood sugar resulting in constantly high levels of insulin.

In 2002, National Institute of Health (NIH) designated Syndrome X as a new target for the prevention of coronary heart disease (CHD). According to NIH's guideline, Syndrome X is diagnosed when three or more of the following factors present:

Risk Factor	Defining Level
• Abdominal Obesity	(Waist Circumference)
Men	>40 in (102cm)
Women	>35 in (88 cm)
• Triglycerides	≥150 mg/dl
• HDL Cholesterol	
Men	<40 mg/dl
Women	<50 mg/dl
• Blood Pressure	≥130/≥85 mmHg
• Fasting Glucose	≥110 mg/dl

2) INSULIN RESISTANCE

Insulin is the hormone secreted by the pancreas that decreases circulating levels of blood sugar (glucose) by facilitating its entry into cells, to be used as energy or stored for later use. Circulating glucose that is not utilized by the cells may be stored as fat throughout the body. Constantly high levels of glucose may increase oxidative stress leading to damage by free radicals. What happens over time with the consumption of refined carbohydrates is that the cells develop a resistance to the body's own insulin. When the cells do not bind with insulin, or the insulin does not "trigger" glucose absorption, it goes back into circulation, re-stimulating the pancreas in its effort to remove the glucose from the bloodstream and get it into the cells to produce even more insulin. As more insulin contacts the cells, they become even more resistant. Imagine this cycle repeating itself over and over, three, four or more times a day, year in and year out. This is the process that sets the stage for the development of Syndrome X and a range of cardiovascular disorders.

Insulin resistance, a prediabetic condition, is at the core of Syndrome X. Under this condition, insulin levels are elevated but glucose levels remain high because cells are desensitized and no longer respond to insulin. Accelerated aging is among the consequences since the high blood sugar levels create more free radicals, which damage DNA.

3) THE NATURAL APPROACH

The good news is that Insulin Resistance and Syndrome X can be prevented and reversed by a combination of diet, moderate physical activity and proper supplementation. Dietary recommendations are not unlike those suggested for other health conditions. It is a diet that would benefit everyone:

Syndrome X Dietary Guidelines
1. Watch your calorie intake.
2. Avoid trans fats and partially hydrogenated oils.

3. Limit saturated fat.
4. Increase omega-3 fatty acids.
5. Reduce intake of sugar and other processed/refined carbohydrates.
6. Consume fiber and/or protein with high-glycemic foods to minimize the spike in blood sugar.

Essential vitamins, minerals, trace elements and antioxidants play key roles in the body's glucose/insulin metabolism and protect against deleterious effects of excess glucose and insulin. Of special importance are alpha-lipoic acid, vitamins E and C and trace mineral chromium. Also, bitter melon, *Gymnema sylvestre* and maitake mushroom have demonstrated blood sugar-lowering effects. However, Maitake SX-Fraction™ is the first proprietary dietary supplement product of its kind in the market with scientific validation targeting Syndrome X.

Before explaining SX-*fraction*'s use against Syndrome X in detail, let's discuss briefly maitake mushroom and its very effective standardized extract, D-*fraction*, which has been in the market since 1995, and has established its credential as a leading immune-boosting product.

Maitake: King of Mushrooms

One of the most delicious and uniquely tasty mushrooms in the world is the maitake mushroom (*Grifola frondosa*). So highly prized as a food that at one time in Japan it was worth its weight in silver. Maitake is a large mushroom, often reaching twenty inches at the base, and a single cluster can weigh as much as one hundred pounds. Its size and amazing health benefits are why it has come to be called "the king of mushrooms." It is the only edible mushroom in the Monkey's bench family, which are well-known immune enhancers.

Several years ago, researchers began to examine and compare a variety of mushrooms traditionally thought of as food with some of the leading mushrooms that have long been employed as medicine. The end result of this research demonstrated that the maitake mushroom had a stronger immune potentiating effect and tumor inhibition rate than any other medicinal mushrooms. The next step was to determine what specifically was in maitake that was stimulating these responses.

D-*fraction:* The Proteoglucan

Researchers found that a unique protein-bound, beta-glucan compound (proteoglucan) in maitake was the strongest immune-boosting component in the mushroom. They called it D-*fraction.* Initial research focused on D-*fraction's* ability to stimulate a variety of immune cell activity, especially certain cytokines (chemical messengers of the immune system). Some of the immune responses include natural killer cells, macrophages, cytotoxic T cells, interleukin 1 and 2 and tumor necrosis factor (TNF)-α.[1] What this means for us is that the D-*fraction* is able to boost the immune system so that there are more immune cells doing more of what immune cells are supposed to be doing. One of the intriguing aspects of this research is that they found D-*fraction* to be almost as effective when used orally as it is when injected.[2] This is significant because far too often research done with injectable forms is then applied to products that are used orally.

It is well known that beta glucan, a complex polysaccharide composed of glucose molecules strung together, is largely responsible for the immune-activating and anti-tumor properties of maitake and some other medicinal mushrooms. Beta-glucans by themselves, however, lose much of their effectiveness when taken orally. Maitake's D-*fraction* is a protein-bound beta glucan (proteoglucan) designed to be effective when taken orally.

In 1995, a dietary supplement product based on this concentrated proteoglucan from maitake mushroom, named Maitake D-Fraction®, was introduced to the U.S. supplement market by Maitake Products, Inc. D-*fraction* has been tested extensively and proven effective in potentiating cellular immune responses, inhibiting carcinogenesis (the creation of cancer)[2] tumor growth and metastasis (the spreading of cancer)[3] and inducing apoptosis (the self-destruction of cancer cells).[4] In a Japanese human clinical trial, it was found to improve the outcome of many types of cancer including breast, lung, liver and prostate, and to enhance chemotherapy treatment while reducing its side effects.[5] (See Figure 1.)

In 1998, the U.S. Food and Drug Administration approved an Investigational New Drug application for Maitake D-Fraction®, making it one of only a few natural products ever to have this authorization for use in clinical trials. (See Woodland Health Series *Maitake Mushroom and D-Fraction* for more information on D-*fraction* and cancer research.)

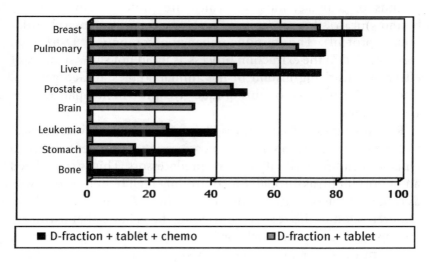

Figure 1.
Improvement Rate in Various Cancers by D-Fraction

SX-*fraction:* The Glycoprotein

The success of D-*fraction* inspired more research to identify other bio-active compounds in maitake. Maitake Products, Inc. has collaborated on studies with Japanese and U.S. researchers on antidiabetic activities of maitake since 1994 and has identified another proteoglucan compound that enhances insulin sensitivity and helps ameliorate diabetic conditions. This active compound was named WS-*fraction* by Dr. Harry Preuss, M.D., Ph.D., a professor of Physiology, Medicine and Pathology at Georgetown University,[6] and has been under the patent in the United States since June 30, 1998 (U.S. Patent #5,773,426).

The WS-*fraction* became the starting material for development of a new, more effective compound called SX-*fraction* (named *grislin* in Japan). During the period of laboratory studies on WS-*fraction* at Georgetown University, Dr. Cun Zhuang, Ph.D., Research and Development at Maitake Products, has successfully come up with this new compound, SX-*fraction*. Unlike previous active compounds of maitake, most of which are proteoglucan (protein-bound glucan), this SX-*fraction* is a glycoprotein (oligosaccharide-bound protein). The immune-enhancing compound, D-*fraction*, was removed in the extraction process as it did not show significant effect of sensitizing insulin in the animal studies at Georgetown. The patent is pending on this unique glycoprotein in Japan and the Unites States.

Recent studies at Georgetown University and New York Medical College confirm that SX-*fraction* possesses a more potent ability to enhance insulin sensitivity than its predecessors. This is considered an important breakthrough for controlling high blood sugar as well as other disorders related to disturbed glucose/insulin metabolism. Dr. Preuss found the research intriguing; he believes that if you are able to restore normal levels of insulin and blood sugar, you can interrupt the pernicious cycle of obesity and age-related disorders collectively known as Syndrome X.

Hypertension

Blood pressure is described as the pressure of the circulating blood on the walls of the arteries. It is maintained by the contractions of the heart, the resistance and elasticity of blood vessels and the volume and viscosity of the blood. The maximum pressure (systolic) occurs at the synchronized contractions of the muscles of the heart chambers. The minimum pressure (diastolic) occurs during relaxation of these muscles at which time the chambers fill with blood. On average, a young adult has a blood pressure of about 120/80. The upper limit of normal blood pressure is considered 140/90.

Hypertension is an intermittent or sustained elevation of blood pressure. In a healthy person, physical activity or emotional tension will cause a temporary rise in pressure which returns to normal after a period of relaxation. It is abnormal when the pressure remains high. High blood pressure without any apparent cause, such as a kidney infection, obstruction of an artery or an adrenal disorder, is referred to as essential or primary hypertension. It is estimated that 15–20 percent of all adults have high blood pressure.

Elevated blood pressure increases the work load on the heart because it is forced to pump against a greater resistance. A constant strain is also placed on the vasculature. In the tiny capillaries of the kidney where pressure is normally high, there is also a risk of damage. For this reason, high blood pressure, if untreated, can cause heart and kidney disease or stroke (obstruction of blood flow to the brain caused by a blood clot).

People who are overweight are good candidates for high blood pressure. Losing weight will reduce the risk. It is estimated that each 10 percent reduction in weight reduces the risk of heart disease by 20 percent due in part to blood pressure normalization.

High blood pressure is not an inevitable part of aging as often thought. There are some populations in which older people have the same blood pressure as the younger ones. Diet appears to be a big factor. Diets of these non-acculturated societies differ from acculturated societies—containing less sodium, simple sugars and saturated fats (meat, butter, whole milk) and containing more complex carbohydrates, fibers and potassium. Exercise also plays an essential role since indigenous cultures tend to live a more rigorous and active lifestyle.

Dr. Preuss' studies show that hypertension and insulin resistance can be produced in rats by heavy feeding on simple sugars. In this animal model, he has found that the most sensitive indicator correlating with increased insulin resistance is a significant elevation of systolic blood pressure.[7]

Hypertension is more prevalent among diabetics. Thus, it is not surprising that measures which enhance insulin sensitivity and ameliorate high blood sugar and high insulin (such as exercise and medication) also lower blood pressure and reduce the risk of other heart and blood vessel risk factors.

Previous studies using whole maitake mushroom powder have demonstrated a blood pressure lowering effect. In a 1987 study, Japanese researchers studied the effect of maitake on hypertension in spontaneously hypertensive rats.[8] The rats were divided into two groups and fed either a normal ration or one containing 5 percent whole mushroom powder. After nine weeks, both blood pressure and very low-density lipoprotein (VLDL) cholesterol dropped in the maitake group.

A study on Zucker Fatty Rats (ZFR), genetically diabetic rats with insulin resistance, was conducted at Georgetown University.[6] The research was conducted for one month, but by fifth day, the systolic blood pressure of the ZFR consuming the diets containing whole maitake powder and WS-*fraction* was already significantly lower than the control group by approximately 15–20 mmHg.

Maitake has played an important role in the practice of Abram Ber, M.D. of Scottsdale, Arizona. He treated over thirty patients with maitake during a period of two to three months. He states, "When on medication, the blood pressure is all over the place, but with maitake mushroom there is a gradual decrease in blood pressure toward normalcy. Further, there are absolutely no side effects." Dr. Ber's treatment program includes three grams of maitake caplets per day for the first week, four grams per day the second week, then five grams per day, adjusting the dosage as the patients' blood pressure readings dictate.

Cholesterol and Triglycerides

High levels of cholesterol and triglycerides are both indicators of increased risk for heart disease and are part and parcel of diabetic- and Syndrome X-related complications. Unfortunately, millions of Americans suffer from high blood levels of cholesterol and triglycerides. While medical drugs may help to reduce cholesterol levels, their side effects may make them less desirable than safe natural medicines.

Health-conscious people recognize that high levels of cholesterol in their blood increase their risk of heart disease. Cholesterol is not a fat but is closely related to it. It is a waxy substance that is an essential component in the structure of cells and is also involved in the formation of adrenal and sex hormones. If your diet contained no cholesterol, your liver would still produce all the cholesterol you need.

However, high levels of a particular kind of cholesterol called low density lipoprotein (LDL, or the so-called "bad cholesterol") and very low density lipoprotein (VLDL or very bad cholesterol) can contribute to coronary artery disease in which the blood vessels are narrowed by deposits of fatty tissue called atheromas, which are made up largely of cholesterol. Narrowing of the heart's coronary arteries by patches of atheroma can cause angina. This also increases the risk of an artery becoming blocked by a blood clot.

On the other hand, your body also produces high density lipoproteins (HDLs, "good cholesterol") which are quickly transported from the bloodstream and do not form atheroma deposits in the arteries. HDL cholesterol also helps your body breakdown the "bad" cholesterol.

What many people don't realize, however, is that triglycerides, a type of fat, are now thought to be an even greater risk factor for heart disease. High levels of triglycerides can influence the size, density, distribution and composition of LDL cholesterol leading to smaller, denser LDL particles which are more likely to promote the obstructions in the blood vessels that trigger heart attack. In a healthy person, triglycerides and other fatty substances are normally moved into the liver and into storage cells to provide energy for later use. Elevated triglycerides can be caused by consuming too much sugar and may be a consequence of other diseases such as diabetes.

Thanks to Quaker Oats, consumers are starting to associate beta glucans with another important health benefit: reducing cholesterol. Over the past three decades, at least thirty-seven separate human studies have demonstrated that oat meal and oat bran can reduce serum cholesterol—even in those consuming a low-fat, low-cholesterol diet. In 1997, an FDA ruling allowed manufacturers to say that soluble fiber from whole oats, oat bran or oat flour as part of a low-saturated fat, low-cholesterol diet may reduce the risk of heart disease.

Chemists have isolated a beta glucan as the key active ingredient for the cholesterol-lowering effect of oat bran. As with other soluble fiber components, the binding of cholesterol (and bile acids) by beta glucans and the resulting elimination of these molecules in the feces is very helpful for reducing blood cholesterol. To be sure, beta glucans found in oats and from yeasts and fungi such as maitake mushroom are not identical. In their natural state, yeast and mushrooms contain a mixture of beta 1,3 glucan and beta 1,6 glucan. Oats and barley contain a mixture of beta 1,3 glucan and beta 1,4 glucan. Yet, both have a beneficial effect on serum lipid levels.[9] Oat beta glucans are found in various breakfast cereals and snacks. Usually, several servings of these products are required to meet the FDA's claim of reducing the risk of heart disease. The yeast- or fungi-derived fiber is a more concentrated source of beta glucan than the oat products. It is also currently being tested in a wide variety of food products for its cholesterol-lowering effects. Thus far, results have been encouraging.

Heart disease is the leading cause of death in the U.S., but one way to reduce the risk of developing the disease is to lower serum cholesterol levels by making dietary changes. In addition to reducing intake of total fat, saturated fat and trans fats, serum cholesterol can be further reduced by adding maitake or its SX-*fraction* to the diet.

In a 1987 experiment at Tohoku University, Japan, with hypertensive rats which were fed: a regular diet, one containing 5 percent shiitake, or one containing 5 percent maitake, the maitake-fed group experienced greater reduction of blood and liver cholesterol and triglyceride levels than the shiitake-fed group or the control group.[10]

Another study conducted at Shizuoka University, Japan, in 1992 also clearly indicated that maitake powder is useful for lowering cholesterol and triglyceride levels.[11] One group of five-week-old rats

Group	Plasma lipid concentration (mg/dl)		
	Cholesterol	Triglyceride	Phospholipid
25 % Casein	364±28	126±10	176±12
25 % Casein + 5% Maitake	274±19	104±6	149±7

	Liver lipid (mg/g)		
	Cholesterol	Triglyceride	Phospholipid
25 % Casein	75.2±0.9	54.3±3.8	26.5±0.3
25 % Casein + 5% Maitake	69.9±1.8	46.6±2.1	25.7±0.3

Table 1.
Antihyperlipemic Effects of Maitake on Rats

was fed a high cholesterol diet and another group was fed the same diet plus 5 percent maitake powder. The results after fourteen days are summarized in Table 1.

These studies suggest that maitake reduces serum lipids and may have cardioprotective effects and reduce the risk of stroke and cardiovascular disease. The usual dosage for this purpose is three to six grams daily of whole maitake powder caplets.

Obesity

Another feature of Syndrome X is abdominal obesity, not overall obesity but specifically the "old spare tire" around the waist. This is determined by waist measurement. A waist circumference of more than thirty-nine inches in men and thirty-four inches for women indicates abdominal obesity. According to WHO's guidance, waist to hip ratio exceeds 1:1 in men and 1:0.85 in women would indicate this type of the obesity.

Most people who are overweight have insulin resistance. There's a bit of a "chicken and egg" argument, though, as to which event happens first. Does being overweight cause insulin resistance or vice versa? One thing we do know is insulin lowers blood sugar (glucose) by facilitating its entry into cells to be used for energy.

Insulin, however, is also a fat storage hormone because it converts glucose ultimately into fat (triglycerides). Because the link between diabetes and obesity is so strong, the combination has been termed "diabesity." It is most likely that each contributes to the other; the more obese one is, the more likely one in insulin resistant; and the more insulin resistant, the greater likelihood of obesity. Like much of the Syndrome X condition, a cycle is created, increasing insulin resistance and obesity "feeding" each other.

High levels of insulin and eventual insulin resistance can be avoided by following the Syndrome X dietary guidelines and including appropriate nutritional supplements. Diabetics or those who present symptoms of Syndrome X may gain improved peripheral insulin sensitization and glycemic control by supplementing with maitake.

Maitake's anti-obesity activity has been studied in both animals and humans. In a 1992 study in Japan, rats were divided into three groups: those fed with normal feed (control), those with 10 percent maitake powder, and those with 20 percent maitake powder. The body weight increase in the 20 percent maitake group only showed 20–30g, while that of control group gained as much as 140 g.[12]

In another study in Japan, the gain of average body weight of rates which were fed high-cholesterol diets containing 5 percent maitake powder during the two weeks of experiment period was 66 g compared to 79 g of gain in control group given high-cholesterol diets only.[11]

At the Koseikai Clinic in Tokyo, Dr. Masanori Yokota, M.D. gave thirty obese patients twenty 500 mg caplets of maitake powder daily for a period of two months with no change in their regular diets.[13] All of the patients lost weight (between seven and twenty-six pounds) with an average loss of eleven to thirteen pounds. Dr. Yokota believes he got better results with this regime than with any other one he had tried and speculates that the patients would have continued to lose weight if the study had continued beyond two months.

Maitake when used as crude powder in caplet form, appears to be a highly effective weight-loss nutrient. However, it must be taken at relatively high doses of about 5–10 grams daily (up to twenty 500 mg caplets). (Note: Even at these dosages, maitake is completely nontoxic.) A good bit of news on the new compound SX-*fraction* is that Japanese clinical study as mentioned later confirmed significant decrease of body weight among type 2 diabetic patients in just two months.

Diabetes

Diabetes mellitus is a disease in which blood levels of glucose (a simple sugar) are abnormally high because the body doesn't release or use insulin adequately. A chronically high blood glucose level in all diabetic patients may cause serious clinical complications and lead to blindness, kidney failure, amputation, coma and death. This metabolic disorder currently affects over 16 million people in the United States and some 250 million people worldwide and is one of the fastest growing diseases.

Diabetes is classified into two types: type 1 (insulin-dependent diabetes) and type 2 (not insulin-dependent). Type 1 diabetes is caused primarily by insulin deficiency and represents less than 20 percent of all cases of diabetes, while type 2 diabetes, with a greater than 80 percent incidence rate, involves multiple factors such as defects in insulin secretion, insulin resistance at peripheral sites (muscle and fat tissue) and elevated liver glucose production. The incidence of type 2 diabetes is often associated with obesity and aging (usually individuals over forty years old), although the exact reason yet remains unknown. Sadly, this seems to be changing with younger and younger people now becoming afflicted with type 2 diabetes.

With regard to treatment, type 1 diabetes is more likely managed through insulin injection than type 2 diabetes since it is linked primarily to pancreatic insulin deficiency. In many type 2 cases, insulin deficiency is not the primary problem, but rather peripheral *insulin resistance* is the major factor for elevated blood sugar conditions. In fact, because of insulin resistance, current oral therapy using medication, which primarily stimulates insulin secretion from pancreatic beta cells, often fails to achieve an expected level of efficacy.

Thus, more effective treatment of type 2 diabetics relies mainly on how to overcome insulin resistance. To enhance peripheral insulin sensitivity, pharmaceuticals such as troglitazone and metformin have been developed. Although these drugs provide some improved glycemic control, there are potential adverse effects. It is rare, but metformin may cause lactic acidosis presenting as impairment of kidney function, shock or liver failure. Due to severe liver toxicity, troglitazone has been removed from the U.S. market. This raises the questions: Are there alternative means to overcome insulin resistance safely? Are any safer *natural* agents available? Such agents could be a key to a better treatment for type 2 diabetics.

Syndrome X and type 2 diabetes have much in common. Both are very complex diseases where insulin deficiency is not typically the problem but insulin resistance is. With insulin resistance, a sufficient amount of insulin is produced by the pancreas, but it is not being used or metabolized properly for glucose uptake in peripheral sites. This results in the build-up of glucose and insulin in the bloodstream. In other words, many people with insulin resistance are prone to the overproduction of insulin, leading to hyperglycemia (high blood sugar) and a high blood insulin level. It is very important that not only blood glucose but also blood insulin should be maintained at the appropriate (normal) levels because disturbances in glucose/insulin metabolism, due principally to insulin resistance, have been shown to hasten the overall aging process. As far as a therapeutic approach is concerned, because Syndrome X occurs in a cluster, taking the steps to bring one of the conditions into a healthy range would subsequently improve the others. However, no specific/effective drugs are available for this syndrome.

In the meantime, the possibility of maitake mushroom as a safe, natural agent for treatment of type 2 diabetes and Syndrome X accompanied by insulin resistance has been examined for the past several years. Several studies show that maitake fractions do have glucose-lowering potential.

A recent study with diabetic mice (KK mice) found that a single, small dose of WS-*fraction* significantly decreased glucose levels up to sixteen hours (Figure 2), thus the dosage of twice or three times a day is suggested.[14]

WS-*fraction* (28 mg/mouse)

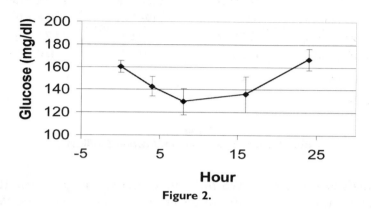

Figure 2.

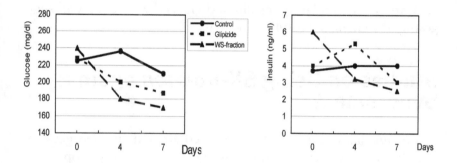

Figure 3.
Antidiabetic Effect of WS-*fraction* on KK-Mice

For comparison, glipizide, an oral diabetic medicine, was also tested. Although there was a nonsignificant trend toward decreased glucose levels, the drug failed to produce significant reductions in glucose and insulin concentrations (Figure 3). The researchers concluded that WS-*fraction* appeared to perform as well as the diabetes drug in a long-term trial.

A similar study using Zucker Fatty Rat (ZFR, a diabetic model with insulin resistance) was also conducted at Georgetown University.[6] The blood chemistry data in control and test rats, hav-

ZFR	Control	Maitake	WS-*fraction*
Glucose (mg/dl)	215±18.8	219±13.4	186±14.0
Insulin (ulU/dl)	78.7±3.7	65.8±6.1*	71.7±3.3#
HbA1C (%)	5.7±0.17	5.1±0.19*	5.4±0.12#

* p < 0.05
# p< 0.10

Table 2.
Blood Chemistries (on WS-*fraction* Studies)

ing maitake powder and WS-*fraction*, respectively is summarized in Table 2. Although a significant effect of maitake powder and WS-*fraction* were not seen on circulating glucose levels, the lower concentrations of circulating insulin and HbA1C were observed, suggesting the enhanced insulin sensitivity.

Studies on Using SX-*fraction* against Syndrome X

Various laboratory studies were conducted at Georgetown University to examine the effects of newly developed glycoprotein from Maitake, SX-*fraction*, against Syndrome X or insulin resistance syndrome.

Dr. Preuss believes that one of the most sensitive indices correlating with increased insulin resistance is a significant elevation of systolic blood pressure (SBP) above baseline. SBP on young ZFR was measured along with body weight and other blood chemistries. In one study, SBP of the control group rose steadily over six weeks from an average of 119 to 150, an increase of 31 points. In contrast, the blood pressure of those fed SX-*fraction* increased significantly less—119 to 125 (Figure 4).[15] In addition, fasting blood glucose was statistically lower in rats given SX-*fraction* (140) as compared to the control group (159) (Table 3).

Another animal study using ZFRs at seventy weeks of age

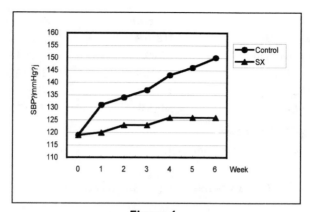

Figure 4.
Antihypertensive Effect of SX-*fraction* on the Young ZFR

Group	Glucose (mg/dl)	Cholesterol (mg/dl)	Triglyceride (mg/dl)	AST (U/L)	ALT (U/L)	Creatinine (mg/dl)	BUN (mg/dl)
Control	159+/-6.5	133+/-12.9	576+/-89	105+/-12.0	84+/-8.9	0.5+/-0.06	15+/-1.2
Test	140+/-4.8	128+/-7.8	453+/-93	95+/-10.9	69+/-6.2	0.4+/-0.07	15+/-1.4

Table 3.
Antidiabetic and Antihyperlipidemic Effects of SX-*fraction* on Young ZFR

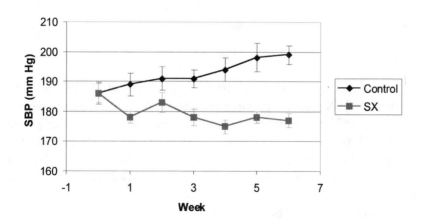

Figure 5.

	Control	SX-*fraction*
Glucose (mg/dl)	218±18	151±11*
Creatinine (mg/dl)	1.3±0.3	1.4±0.8
BUN (mg/dl)	41±10.2	39±18.5
ALT (U/L)	56±3.6	79±10.4
AST (U/L)	54±5.8	55±7.2

Average + SEM shown

* Significantly different from control

Table 4.
Blood Chemistries (on SX-*fraction* Study)

Aging Studies

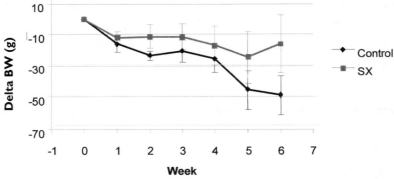

Figure 6.

demonstrated even more drastic results.[16] The initial SBP for both control and SX-*fraction* group were about 185 mmHg. In six weeks, the SBP of SX group decreased to 176, while that for control group increased to almost 200 (Figure 5). Also, the blood glucose for the SX group (151 mg/al) was significantly lower compared to that for control group (218 mg/al) (Table 4). Researchers concluded that SX-*fraction* significantly lowers systolic blood pressure and fasting blood sugar and may be useful in treating insulin resistance.

Further, this study was performed by Dr. Preuss at Georgetown

University using an older group of obese and diabetic rats that were entering the last stages of life.[16] These rats were in declining health with a rapid loss in body weight. It is observed that when those rats were force-fed SX-*fraction*, overall health was enhanced without the loss of body weight (Figure 6). Dr. Preuss concluded that this result demonstrates that elderly diabetics and aging individuals with insulin resistance might benefit from SX-*fraction*.

Clinical Cases

A) A STUDY ON DIABETIC PATIENTS IN THE U.S.

In a clinical study, five volunteer patients with type 2 diabetes taking oral medication demonstrated improved blood sugar levels with maitake mushroom powder (MMP) caplets containing the active component with hypoglycemic activity (SX-*fraction*).[17, 18] There was a decline of 30–63 percent in their blood glucose levels in two to four weeks. One patient showed complete glycemic control and is currently free of medications. Table 5 summarizes the hypoglycemic effects of MMP on diabetic patients.

A seventy-five-year-old woman in the study had type 2 diabetes for six years. Her average fasting blood glucose (FBG) level was around 200 mg/dl with a glycosylated hemoglobin (HbA) level of

Patients	Age (yr)	Sex	Average FBG (mg/dL)		Percent of FBG declined with MPC
			Before MMP	After MMP	
A	44	M	~260	90~100	~63
B	75	F	~200	11~130	~40
C	25	F	150~180	110~120	~30
D	37	M	180~200	120~140	~32
E	43	M	~220	100~110	~52

Table 5.
Summary of Hypoglycemic Effects of MMP on Diabetic Patients

9.1 percent under daily glyburide (5 mg) therapy. Once she was placed on 3 MMPs per day with glyburide, her FBG began declining and remained at 110–130 for the next 2-1/2 months. Glyburide was then reduced to 2.5 mg with MMPs, and her current FBG is less than 130.

While this trial was small, the body of maitake research over the last fifteen years makes it reasonable to say that diabetics or those with Syndrome X may gain improved peripheral insulin sensitization and glycemic control by supplementing with SX-*fraction*. Numerous human and animal studies have demonstrated that whole maitake or its fractions are potent agents for improving "diabetic conditions." Maitake SX-*fraction* is the culmination of this research.

B) ANOTHER STUDY IN JAPAN

In June 2003, the first international seminar to discuss Syndrome X among researchers and medical doctors from the United States and Japan was held in Tokyo, Japan. The result of a two-month clinical study using SX-*fraction* on fourteen type 2 diabetes patients was presented (Figures 7 and 8). Although preliminary, researchers confirm the following findings from the study:

1. Fasting blood glucose and hemoglobin A1C decreased in a month with statistical significance.

Effects on Glucose Metabolism

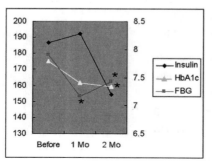

Effects on Lipid Metabolism

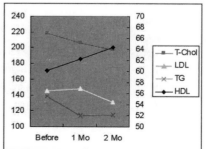

Figure 7.

Figure 8.

2. There was a steady and statistically significant decrease in body weight.
3. Total and LDL cholesterols as well as triglyceride showed tendency to decrease.
4. HDL cholesterol seemed to increase, and insulin to decrease.

A Testimonial for Hyperglycemia

Dr. Konno, a researcher heavily involved with maitake study and co-author of *Maitake Magic* (Freedom Press, 2002), gives his personal history of being diagnosed with diabetes as follows:

"I am an Associate Professor and a Research Director of Urology at New York Medical College. The main theme of my research focuses on urological cancer, particularly on prostate cancer. Unfortunately, conventional treatments for prostate cancer are currently rather ineffective and finding/establishing more effective treatments is urgently demanded.

"Going back to the early summer of 1999 when we were conducting a maitake D-fraction study on prostate cancer, it turned out to be the year for me to remember. I had begun to notice that I was hungry and felt thirsty quite often and then started going to the bathroom more frequently. I must have drunk tons of water and went to the bathroom many times a day! Concurrently, I started losing weight rapidly. I was overweight, usually weighing around 185 pounds for only 5'7" tall, but my weight had gone down to 155, a loss of 30 pounds in about two months. However, frequent thirst and urination and drastic weight-loss are typical signs of hyperglycemia (high blood glucose) or type 2 diabetes.

"As I expected, a simple blood test revealed that my fasting blood glucose (FBG) level was nearly 248 mg/dl, which was much higher than the normal upper level of 115. Another blood test showed my glycosylated hemoglobin (HbAlc) level was 11.5 percent which was also higher than the normal range of 5–7.5 percent. These two blood parameters confirmed or most likely indicated that I might have become diabetic. Fortunately, no retinopathy/neuropathy or diabetes-related complications had yet developed. I was thus diagnosed with early stage type 2 diabetes at the age of 44.

"Coincidentally, I had learned that the company providing us D-fraction for the prostate cancer study happened to have another maitake mushroom product with blood glucose-lowering (hypoglycemic) activity. This unique product was referred to as 'fraction SX' which was initially only available in a 500 mg caplet of maitake mushroom powder (MMP). SX-Fraction™ (Maitake Products, Inc.), a highly purified form of MMP, has become commercially available this year (2003).

"Now, as soon as my diagnosis was made, I was immediately given daily 2.5 mg oral glyburide therapy and my FBG level went down from 248 to 180 over the next 2 days. I also started taking a 500 mg MMP caplet three times per day with glyburide on the third day. (Note: the reason I took MMP was that SX-Fraction™ was not yet available at the time.) My FBG on the next day had declined to 83, followed by a quick rise to approximately 120 and then a gradual decrease to roughly 100 in ten days. After this short adjustment period, my FBG levels remained 80–90 mg/dl for the next three months and HbAlc was also down to 5.2 percent. Glyburide was then reduced to 1.25 mg with two MMP a day, and my FBG levels still remained 80–90 mg/dl for the next two months. Consequently, glyburide was completely withdrawn but I was kept on daily MMPs two times per day, and my FBG levels remained at approximately 90 and my HbAlc remained at 5.6 percent over six months. Now, it has been over four years since my initial diagnosis, but I am currently free of any medications except for 2 MMPs/day and remain normoglycemic.

"Although the mechanism of hypoglycemic action of 'fraction SX' is not fully defined, it is postulated that such an active maitake fraction may, in part, enhance peripheral insulin sensitivity, thereby weakening insulin resistance.

"As I mentioned earlier, MMP was used as a source of fraction SX with hypoglycemic activity in my case study. I am sure that SX-fraction, a highly purified form of MMP now available, should be highly potent and more effective on glycemic control of diabetic patients, although more valid clinical data are yet required. Nevertheless, I recently started taking SX-Fraction™ instead of MMP and all my physiological parameters remain normal. Of course, most importantly I have not experienced any side effects related to this product. I personally believe that SX-Fraction™ is indeed a safe product to be consumed by everyone.

Particularly, people with type 2 diabetes may gain great benefits from this unique fraction, and so it would be worthwhile trying it.

"In addition, SX-Fraction™ is claimed to help lose body weight. Several cases of volunteers who took SX-Fraction™ for weight-loss showed some promising results after their two-month trial. Therefore, it is very interesting and valuable to carry out more trials to properly evaluate its potential weight-loss effect.

"Lastly, I hope this personal story might encourage those suffering from type 2 diabetes and help them find a better way to cope with it."

Another Testimonial for Hypoglycemia

Let me also introduce an exciting testimonial from another supporter of SX-*fraction*, Dr. Elisa Lotter. Dr. Elisa Lotter is a board-certified naturopathic physician and an HMD (homeopathic medical doctor) with a Ph.D. in Nutrition. She has been in private practice in Southern California for the past twenty years, integrating preventative health and natural medicine into her practice. For the last few years, she has been warning the American public that there is a silent epidemic which spans all age groups, from children to baby boomers to seniors; it is hypoglycemia or low blood sugar. She claims that many women beginning menopause will have a large percentage of the symptoms, such as fatigue, dizziness, headache, depression, anxiety, night sweats, swollen feet, insomnia, etc. But this is not a woman's syndrome only and many men also exhibit these symptoms.

Hypoglycemia may be another case of malfunction of insulin/glucose metabolism, where an abnormally low level of glucose stays in the blood. Obviously, this is not caused by a state of insulin resistance, as hypoglycemia often results from the over-secretion of insulin.

She has a number of nutritional regimens to prevent or treat this health problem and has the following special comment on maitake or SX-*fraction*:

"Although conventional nutritional research cites a number of supplements reputed to be efficacious in managing or treating this condi-

tion such as: chromium, L-Glutamine, licorice, vanadyl sulfate, bitter melon, cinnamon bark, etc., which I have used in my practice for over twenty years, I have not found any to be as successful as the maitake SX-fraction. I have found in case after case that this product is invaluable not only for prevention, but also for treating those suffering from chronic hypoglycemia."

How to Take Maitake SX-Fraction™

The recommended dose of SX-Fraction™ for Syndrome X is one tablet, three times per day within thirty minutes after meals. The clinical protocol for diabetics is two to three tablets, three times daily. This might be necessary to continue two months or more in order to experience the full therapeutic potential. After the effects have stabilized, the dose is reduced to a maintenance amount, one to two tablets, three times daily. Note: SX-Fraction™ was developed with type 2 diabetes and Syndrome X in mind, but it is possible that it may also help type 1 (insulin-dependent). Interestingly, most of the people who participated in the clinical studies have reported significant improvement of their abdominal obesity as a pleasant side effect.

Cautions and Safety

While maitake has a long history of safety, if you are taking prescription medication for diabetes, consult your doctor before taking any dietary supplement or changing your diet. Your blood sugar should be monitored carefully since supplements can make your medicine dangerously potent. An FDA-approved investigational new drug application bypassed Phase-1 toxicological studies because of maitake's history of safety. Also, Japan Food Research Laboratories (authorized by The Japanese Government) carried out an LD50 toxicology test on SX-*fraction* and confirmed its safety for clinical use by human.

References

1. Zhuang, C., et al. "Biological Responses from *Grifola frondosa* (Dick.: Fr.) S. F. Gray–Maitake (Aphyllophoromycetideae)." *International Journal of Medicinal Mushrooms*, Vol. 1, pp.317–324 (1999).
2. Lieberman, S. & Babal, K., *Maitake: King of Mushrooms*. Keats Publishing, New Canaan, Connecticut, 1997, p.18.
3. Babal, K. "The cancer-fighting qualities of mushrooms." *Nutrition Science News*. 2(3), 141–2, 1997.
4. Konno, S., et al. "Induction of apoptosis in human prostatic cancer cells with B-glucan (maitake mushroom polysaccharide)." *Molecular Biol*. Vol.4, No.1, 7–13, 2000.
5. Jones, K. "Maitake: A potent medicinal food." *Alternative and Complimentary Therapies*. Dec 1998.
6. Preuss, H., et al. "Antihypertensive and metabolic effects of whole Maitake mushroom powder and its fractions in two rat strains." *Molecular and Cellular Biochemistry*. 237, 129–136, 2002.
7. Preuss, H. et al. "Effect of chromium and guar on sugar-induced hypertension in rats." *Clin Neph*. 1995; 44: 170–177.
8. Kimura, S., et al. "Effect of Shiitake (*Lentinus edodes*) and Maitake (*Grifola frondosa*) Mushrooms on Blood Pressure and Plasma Lipids of Spontaneously Hypertensive Rats." *Nutr. Sci. Vitaminol*. 33, 341–346, 1987.
9. Bell, S., et al. "Effect of beta glucan from oats and yeast on serum lipids." *Crit Rev Food Sci Nutr*. 1999; 39(2): 189–202.
10. Kimura, K., et al. "Effects of shiitake and maitake on plasma cholesterol and blood pressure." *Medicinal Effects of Edible Mushrooms*, Tohoku Univ & Mushroom Institute of Japan, 1–10, Mar 1988.
11. Sugiyama K., et al. "Hypocholesterolemic Activity of Ningyotake (*polyporus confluens*) Mushroom in Rats." *Nihon Eiyo Shokuryo Gakkaishi*. 45(3), 265–270 (1992).
12. Ohtsuru, M. "Anti-obesity activity exhibited by orally administered powder of maitake (*Grifola frondosa*)." *Anshin*. 188–200, July 1992.
13. Yokota, M. "Observatory trial of anti-obesity activity of maitake (*Grifola frondosa*)." *Anshin*. 202–204, July 1992.
14. Manohar, V., et al. "Effects of a water-soluble extract of maitake mushroom on circulating glucose/insulin concentrations in KK mice." *Diabetes, Obesity and Metabolism*. 4, 2002, 43–48.
15. Nadeem, T., et al. "Effects of maitake mushroom fractions on blood pressure of Zucker Fatty Rats." (accepted).
16. Nadeem, T., et al. "Effects of niacin-bound chromium, Maitake mushroom fraction SX and (-)-Hydrozycitric acid on the metabolic syndrome in aged diabetic Zucker fatty rats." (accepted).
17. Konno, S., et al. "A possible hypoglycemic effect of maitake mushroom on type 2 diabetic patients." *Diabetic Med*. 18, 2001.
18. Konno, S., et al. "Anticancer and Hypoglycemic Effects of Polysaccharides in Edible and Medicinal Maitake Mushroom." *International Journal of Medicinal Mushrooms*. Vol. 4, pp. 185–195 (2002).

ABOUT THE AUTHORS

Mark J. Kaylor, Ph.D., M.H., is a holistic healing practitioner and educator in southern California. He has worked at a variety of levels in retail, consulted with companies in formulating products and provided herbal training and formulas for national herbal extract manufacturers. Mark approaches healing from an eclectic and truly holistic point of view, having studied (and continuing to study) many different healing styles and techniques, including American Indian and Traditional Chinese Medicine. Formal education includes BA studies in sociology, AA work in exercise physiology, MA and PhD work in the sociology of change and healing. In his efforts to share the gift and process of healing he has lectured internationally, written numerous articles, appeared on radio and television and has recently started a newsletter, *Talking Trees*. He may be contacted at: talkingtrees@earthlink.net.

Ken Babal is a certified licensed nutritionist through American Health Science University and a member of the Society of Certified Nutritionists. He has a clinical nutrition practice in Los Angeles and is staff nutritionist for Erewhon Natural Foods Market. His articles have appeared in numerous publications including *Nutrition Science News*, *Let's Live*, *Great Health* and *Health Store News*, and has been quoted in others including *The Los Angeles Times*. Ken is an author of *Good Digestion: Your Key to Vibrant Health* (Alive, 2000) and co-author with Shari Lieberman, Ph.D. of *Maitake Mushroom and D-fraction* (Woodland, 2001). He appears in the Discovery Health Channel documentary *Alternatives Uncovered* and E! TV's *High Price of Fame: Starved.*

Woodland Health Series

*Definitive Natural Health Information
At Your Fingertips!*

The Woodland Health Series offers a comprehensive array of single topic booklets, covering subjects from fibromyalgia to green tea to acupressure. If you enjoyed this title, look for other WHS titles at your local health-food store, or contact us. Complete and mail (or fax) us the coupon below and receive the complete Woodland catalog and order form—free!

Or . . .

- Call us toll-free at (800) 777-2665
- Visit our website
  (www.woodlandpublishing.com)
- Fax the coupon (and other correspondence) to
  (801) 785-8511

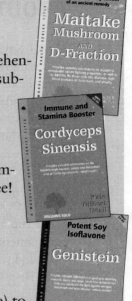